DIVERTICULATIS DIET PLAN GUIDE BOOK

The Complete Diverticulitis Diet Plan for Wellness: Foods that Heal and Soothe Diverticulitis

LARRY HERMAN

Table of Contents

Introduction

Diverticula, which are tiny pouches that can form in the colon's walls, can become inflamed or infected when a person has diverticulitis. When fecal matter becomes stuck in these pouches, it can inflame and cause symptoms including bloating, stomach pain, and altered bowel patterns.

Dietary changes are a common part of diverticulitis management, as they help reduce symptoms and stop flare-ups. Generally speaking, the diverticulitis diet emphasizes easing digestive system discomfort, lowering inflammation, and encouraging bowel regularity.

Important Elements Of A Diet For Diverticulitis Could Be:

• **High-Fiber Foods:** Eating a diet high in fiber helps encourage regular bowel movements and soften stools, which lowers the chance of inflamed diverticula. Good sources of fiber include whole grains, legumes, fruits, and vegetables.

• **Hydration:** Keeping your body well hydrated is essential to preserving intestinal regularity. Constipation is one of the factors that might lead to diverticulitis, so it's important to drink enough water to avoid it.

• Foods low in residue during flare-ups: A low-residue diet may be advised when symptoms of diverticulitis are at their peak. This entails eating meals that are easy on the digestive tract, like refined carbohydrates, lean protein, and well-cooked vegetables.

• **Probiotics:** Adding probiotics to their diet has helped some people feel better. Probiotics are good bacteria that can support gut balance maintenance.

• **Restricting Specific Foods:** It's usually recommended to avoid foods like popcorn, seeds, and nuts that can irritate the digestive system, particularly when flare-ups are occurring.

Diverticulitis sufferers should collaborate closely with medical doctors or a trained dietitian to customize their diet to meet their specific demands and the severity of their illness. Appropriate food selections can be very helpful in controlling diverticulitis and enhancing digestive health in general.

CHAPTER ONE
Diverticulitis: What Is It?

A medical disorder known as diverticulitis affects the colon or large intestine's walls, causing inflammation or infection of tiny pouches called diverticula. These pouches develop when the colon's inner lining pushes outward due to weak spots in the muscle wall. Diverticulitis is a condition that develops when these diverticula become inflamed or infected. Diverticulosis, the condition in which these pouches are present, is typically benign and asymptomatic.

The Following Are Salient Features Of Diverticulitis:

1. Formation of Diverticula: The lining of the digestive system, particularly the colon, can develop tiny, protruding pouches called diverticula. They are more prevalent in older adults and are frequently linked to a diet poor in fiber.

2. Causes: Diverticulitis's precise etiology is unknown, however it is thought to be related to things like a diet low in fiber, which can promote constipation and raise intestinal pressure. Age, inactivity, and genetic factors could also be involved.

3. Diverticulitis symptoms might vary, but they frequently include tenderness, fever, nausea, vomiting, and changes in bowel habits in addition to lower abdomen pain, which is typically on the left side. Diverticulitis can occasionally result in problems like the creation of an abscess, a perforation, or the production of fistulas.

4. Diagnosis: A combination of the patient's medical history, a physical examination, and diagnostic testing is usually used to diagnose diverticulitis. To determine the severity of diverticulitis and to confirm its presence, imaging procedures like CT scans are frequently used.

5. Treatment: Dietary modifications, such as a high-fiber diet to encourage regular bowel movements, may be used to manage mild cases of diverticulitis. Infections are frequently treated with antibiotic prescriptions. In hospitalization, intravenous antibiotics, and sometimes surgical intervention are necessary for severe illnesses or complications.

6. Prevention: Diverticulitis can be avoided by eating a diet high in fiber, drinking plenty of water, and leading a healthy lifestyle. Frequent physical activity and abstaining from risk factors like smoking could aid in prevention.

For a correct diagnosis and course of treatment, it's critical that anyone exhibiting symptoms suggestive of diverticulitis, such as ongoing abdominal pain or changes in bowel habits, seek medical assistance. Complications can be avoided and symptoms can be managed with early management.

A Synopsis of Diverticulitis

A medical illness known as diverticulitis is typified by the development of tiny pouches called diverticula in the walls of the colon or large intestine, which become inflamed or infected. The colon's muscular wall has weak places that cause the inner lining to protrude outward, forming these pouches. Diverticulosis is the term for the presence of diverticula, which are usually innocuous. Diverticulitis, however, results from inflammation or infection of these pouches.

The Following Summarizes The Main Features Of Diverticulitis:

1. Comparing Diverticulitis with Diverticulosis

- **Diverticulosis:** Denotes the existence of diverticula in the absence of infection or inflammation. Diverticulosis may not cause any symptoms in many cases.

- **Diverticulitis**: Caused by inflamed or infected diverticula, this illness manifests as fever, altered bowel habits, stomach pain, tenderness, and occasionally even an abscess or colon perforation.

2. Reasons:

• Although the precise etiology of diverticulitis remains unclear, it is thought to be related to elements including aging, a low-fiber diet, and inactivity. Diets low in fiber can exacerbate constipation by raising colonic pressure and possibly causing diverticula to form.

3. Signs:

• Diverticulitis is commonly characterized by lower abdominal pain, typically on the left side, as well as soreness, fever, nausea, vomiting, and altered bowel patterns. Complications including abscesses, perforations, or fistulas may arise in extreme situations.

4. Conclusion:

• A combination of the patient's medical history, physical examination, and diagnostic tests is usually used to make the diagnosis. Diverticulitis can be diagnosed and its severity evaluated with imaging techniques like CT scans.

5. Therapy:

• Modest cases of diverticulitis can be controlled with dietary modifications, such as consuming a diet rich in fiber to encourage regular bowel movements. Infection-related cases of diverticulitis frequently require the prescription of antibiotics.

• Hospitalization, intravenous antibiotics, and occasionally surgical intervention to treat complications including abscesses or perforations may be necessary in severe cases or complications.

6. Avoidance:

• Diverticulitis can be avoided by following a healthy lifestyle, eating a high-fiber diet, and drinking plenty of water. Preventive measures may also include regular exercise and abstaining from certain risk factors, such as smoking.

For an accurate diagnosis and course of treatment, it's critical that anyone exhibiting symptoms suggestive of diverticulitis seek medical help as soon as possible. Depending on the severity of the symptoms and the existence of complications, the treatment plan may change.

CHAPTER TWO
Reasons and Danger Elements

Diverticulitis' precise causes are unknown, however some circumstances and elements are thought to have a role in its onset. A low-fiber diet is the main factor linked to the development of diverticula and the risk of diverticulitis. The following are some risk factors and causes:

1. Low-Fiber Nutrition:

• One of the main risk factors for diverticulitis is a diet deficient in fiber. Dietary fiber deficiency can cause hard, dry stools and constipation, which can put strain on the colon and encourage the development of diverticula.

2. Growing Older:

• Older persons, especially those over 50, are more likely to get diverticulitis. Diverticula are more likely to form as people age.

3. Absence of Exercise:

• An elevated risk of diverticulitis has been linked to sedentary lifestyles and irregular physical activity. Regular bowel motions and general digestive health can be supported by exercise.

4. Genetic Elements:

• Diverticulitis may have a hereditary component to its development. People who have a family history of the illness can be more vulnerable.

5. Overweight:

• It has been determined that obesity may provide a risk for diverticulitis. Having too much weight on one's frame could raise colonic pressure.

6. Smoking:

• There is evidence that smoking increases the risk of diverticulitis. It is seen as a modifiable risk factor, and the risk could be decreased by giving up smoking.

7. Specific Drugs:

• There may be a higher chance of diverticulitis or related problems if certain drugs, like steroids, opioids, and nonsteroidal anti-inflammatory drugs (NSAIDs), are taken.

8. Former Case of Diverticulosis

• Diverticulitis can occur in those who already have diverticulosis if the diverticula become inflamed or infected.

It's crucial to remember that although diverticulitis may be more common in those who don't seem to have any risk factors, the illness can nonetheless strike healthy people. Furthermore, diverticulitis is not a common side effect of diverticulosis.

A high-fiber diet, frequent exercise, and quitting smoking are all part of a healthy lifestyle that can help reduce some of the risk factors for diverticulitis. It is recommended for people to seek the correct examination and help from a healthcare professional if they have symptoms or have concerns regarding their digestive health.

Signs and Prognosis

Diverticulitis Symptoms Can Differ In Intensity, And Some People With Diverticulosis May Not Exhibit Any Symptoms At All. The Following Signs And Symptoms Of Diverticulitis Could Be Present:

1. Pain in the Abdomen:

• Abdominal pain, usually felt on the lower left side of the abdomen, is a typical sign of diverticulitis. The pain may be slight to severe and may last for a long time.

2. Sensitivity:

- The Abdomen's Afflicted Region Could Become Sensitive To Touch.

3. Colds and Fever:

- Fever and chills are examples of systemic symptoms that can result from an infection or inflammation.

4. Alterations in Bowel Habits

- Bowel Habits Changes, Such as Diarrhea Or Constipation, Can Be Brought On By Diverticulitis.

5. Vomiting and Nauseous:

• Some People Might Feel Queasy Or Throw Up.

6. Gas and Bloating:

• Bloating And Increased Gas May Happen.

7. Bleeding in the Rectal Area:

• Rectal Bleeding is a Possible Side Effect of Diverticulitis, Albeit It Is More Frequently Linked To Diverticulosis.

8. Problems:

• Severe diverticulitis cases or its complications, such as the creation of an abscess, a perforation, or the formation of a fistula, can produce additional symptoms and necessitate prompt medical attention.

Diverticulitis Diagnosis:

1. Medical Background and Physical Assessment:

• To determine the patient's diverticulitis symptoms and indicators, the medical professional will ask about the patient's past medical history and perform a physical examination.

2. Blood Examinations:

• Blood Tests can be Performed to look for Infection-Related Symptoms Including An Increased White Blood Cell Count.

3. Imaging Research:

• Imaging Studies are frequently used to evaluate the severity of diverticulitis and confirm the diagnosis. Typical imaging investigations consist of:

• The CT scan is an essential diagnostic instrument that offers comprehensive images of the abdominal region and detects indications of infection or inflammation.

• **Abdominal Ultrasound:** If CT Scanning is Not Practical; An Ultrasound May Be Used in Certain Situations.

4. Colonoscopy:

- Although a colonoscopy is not usually done while diverticulitis is acute, it might be later on to determine the severity of the disease and rule out other illnesses.

5. Stool Examinations:

- To rule out other potential causes of gastrointestinal problems, such as infections, stool tests may be performed.

The proper management of diverticulitis depends on an accurate and timely diagnosis. People who experience symptoms including fever, altered bowel habits, or ongoing stomach pain should contact a doctor.

A medical expert will carry out the required assessments to identify the root cause of the symptoms and create a suitable treatment strategy.

CHAPTER THREE
Diet's Part in Diverticulitis

Diverticulitis must be managed and prevented in large part through diet. Making certain dietary decisions can aid in symptom relief, lower the chance of problems, and improve digestive health in general. The following are important facets of how nutrition affects diverticulitis:

1. High-Fibre Diet:

• A diet rich in fiber is frequently advised in order to manage and prevent diverticulitis. Fiber gives the feces more volume, which facilitates passage and lowers the chance of constipation. Legumes, whole grains, fruits, and vegetables are all excellent providers of fiber.

2. Fiber, both Soluble and Insoluble:

• Fibers, both soluble and insoluble, support a healthy digestive system. Foods high in soluble fiber, such as fruits, beans, and oats, can aid in softening stools. Vegetables, whole grains, and wheat bran include insoluble fiber, which helps to maintain regular bowel motions by giving the stool more volume.

3. Fluid Consumption:

• Drinking enough water is crucial while consuming more fiber. Water consumption facilitates the passage of fiber through the digestive system and helps avoid constipation.

4. Steer Clear of Specific Foods During Flare-ups:

• A low-residue or low-fiber diet may be advised when diverticulitis symptoms are present in order to lessen the strain on the digestive system. This can entail staying away from roughage, seeds, nuts, and other high-fiber meals in favor of refined carbohydrates, lean protein, and well-cooked veggies.

5. Probiotics:

• Probiotics are good bacteria that can support the gut's ability to remain in a balanced state. Some people find that taking probiotic supplements or consuming foods high in probiotics, like yogurt with living cultures, helps them feel better.

6. Cutting Back on Processed Foods and Red Meat:

• A diet heavy in processed foods and red meat may raise your risk of diverticulitis, according to some research. It could be advantageous to consume more plant-based foods and lean protein sources.

7. Limiting Coffee and Alcohol Use:

• The digestive tract may get irritated by excessive alcohol and caffeine consumption. It may be best to consume alcoholic and caffeinated beverages in moderation.

8. Customized Method:

• Dietary guidelines might differ from person to person, therefore it's important to take tolerances and preferences into account. Dietary recommendations can be more specifically tailored to meet needs when working with a certified dietitian or other healthcare provider.

It's crucial to remember that although nutrition can have a big impact, managing diverticulitis involves other factors as well. The general health of the digestive system is also influenced by lifestyle choices including quitting smoking, eating a healthy weight, and exercising frequently.

Diverticulitis and diverticulosis sufferers should speak with medical professionals to develop a customized diet plan based on their unique symptoms, nutritional requirements, and state of health.

Building a Diverticulitis-Friendly Diet

Building a diverticulitis-friendly diet involves making choices that support digestive health, reduce inflammation, and help prevent flare-ups. Here are general guidelines for creating a diet that may be beneficial for individuals with diverticulitis:

1. High-Fiber Foods: To encourage regular bowel movements and ward off constipation, including a range of high-fiber foods. Fruits (such as apples, pears, and berries) Vegetables (such as leafy greens, carrots, and broccoli) Whole grains (such as oats, whole wheat, and quinoa) and legumes (such as lentils, chickpeas, and black beans) are good sources of fiber.

2. Soluble Fiber: Make sure to eat foods high in soluble fiber, like: oats and oat bran; apples, berries, and citrus fruits; beans and lentils

3. Lean Protein: Add lean protein sources such fish, eggs, skinless chicken, and plant-based proteins (legumes, tofu).

4. Low-Fat Dairy: Choose dairy products that are either low-fat or fat-free, such Greek yogurt.

Moderate amounts of cheese and low-fat milk

5. Good Fats: Select healthy fat sources, such as nuts and seeds, avocado, olive oil, and avocado (in moderation).

6. Fluids: Drink lots of water throughout the day to stay well-hydrated. Consuming enough fluids aids in avoiding constipation.

7. Probiotic-Rich Foods: To promote gut health, think about including foods high in probiotics. A few examples are: yogurt infused with living organisms.

Kefir and fermented foods such as kimchi and sauerkraut

8. Limit Red Meat And Processed Meals: Since they may aggravate inflammation, cut back on your intake of red meat and processed meals. Put more of an emphasis on lean and plant-based protein sources.

9. Moderate Caffeine and Alcohol Intake: Restrict your caffeine and alcohol intake as too much of either might aggravate your digestive tract.

10. Low-Residue Food When There Is A Flare-Up: To give the digestive system a vacation when diverticulitis symptoms are at their worst, think about adopting a low-residue or low-fiber diet. This can include cooked veggies, fruits that have been peeled and refined grains.

It's crucial to remember that everyone has a different tolerance for different foods. It's important to pay attention to individual sensitivities because some people may find that eating specific meals causes symptoms. A licensed dietician or other healthcare expert can offer tailored advice based on each person's unique health needs and preferences.

Furthermore, it's important to gradually modify your diet to give your digestive system time to adjust.

It's critical to get medical guidance for appropriate evaluation and management if symptoms intensify or continue.

The Benefits of Foods High with Fiber

Foods high in fiber are essential for maintaining digestive health in particular and for boosting general health. The following are some major arguments in favor of consuming foods high in fiber in the diet:

1. Encourages Regular Bowel Movements: Dietary fiber gives stool more volume, which softens and makes it simpler to transit through the digestive system. This encourages regular bowel motions and lessens the likelihood of constipation.

2. Prevents and Relieves Constipation: By accelerating the passage of food through the digestive tract, insoluble fiber, which is present in foods like whole grains and vegetables, helps prevent and alleviate constipation.

3. Promotes Digestive Health: A healthy digestive system is mostly dependent on fiber. It helps to prevent a number of gastrointestinal problems, such as hemorrhoids, diverticulitis, and irritable bowel syndrome (IBS).

4. Reduces incidence of Diverticulitis: A diet rich in fiber is linked to a decreased incidence of diverticulitis. Consuming enough fiber helps lower the risk of inflammation and infection as well as the development of diverticula, which are tiny pouches in the colon.

5. Controls Blood Sugar Levels: By reducing the rate at which glucose is absorbed, soluble fiber, which is present in foods like oats and lentils, can help control blood sugar levels. Those who have diabetes would especially benefit from this.

6. Lowers Cholesterol Levels: Research has indicated that soluble fiber can assist in reducing low-density lipoprotein, or LDL, cholesterol levels. This can lower the risk of heart disease and improve cardiovascular health.

7. Encourages Weight Management: Foods high in fiber have fewer calories and make you feel fuller, so they can help regulate appetite and aid in weight management.

8. Promotes Gut Microbiota: o Fiber acts as a prebiotic, giving good gut bacteria energy. Numerous health advantages, such as immune system support and vitamin manufacturing, are linked to a healthy gut flora.

9. Lowers the Chance of Colorectal Cancer: Research has shown that eating enough fiber lowers the chance of developing colorectal cancer. Because fiber reduces colon inflammation and encourages regular bowel movements, it may help guard against this kind of cancer.

10. Enhances Cardiovascular Health: Enhancing heart health and reducing cholesterol levels together lead to better cardiovascular health. A high-fiber diet can help lower the chance of developing heart disease.

It's crucial to remember that the digestive system needs time to adjust, thus boosting fiber intake should be done gradually in addition to drinking enough water. For individualized nutritional advice, people with certain medical issues or concerns should speak with medical specialists or licensed dietitians.

CHAPTER FOUR
Soluble vs. Insoluble Fiber Types

Soluble and insoluble fibers are the two primary categories into which dietary fiber can be roughly divided. Both varieties support the general health of the digestive system and provide unique health advantages. Below is a summary of each:

1. Soluble Fiber:

• **Properties**: Easily dissolved in water, forming a gel-like substance Frequently present in fruit and vegetable flesh, oats, beans, lentils, and some grains.

Health Advantages:

- **Cholesterol Reduction:** By attaching to cholesterol molecules and assisting in their removal from the body, soluble fiber can help lower LDL (low-density lipoprotein) cholesterol levels.

- **Blood Sugar Regulation:** It lowers blood sugar levels by slowing down the absorption of glucose. Those who have diabetes would especially benefit from this.

- **Weight Management:** Soluble fiber increases feelings of fullness and may help control weight by lowering caloric intake in general.

2. Intractable Fiber:

• Its characteristics include adding weight to the stool and resisting dissolving in water.

• Found in whole grains, nuts, seeds, and the skins of fruits and vegetables.

• **Health Benefits:** Encourages Regular Bowel Movement: Insoluble fiber gives stool more volume, which accelerates its passage through the digestive tract and keeps constipation at bay.

• **Colon Health:** It can help avert certain gastrointestinal problems by encouraging regular bowel movements and keeping the colon healthy, such as diverticulosis and hemorrhoids.

- **Weight Management**: Similar to soluble fiber, insoluble fiber also promotes fullness, which helps control weight by preventing overindulgence.

3. Foods High in Soluble Fiber: - Oats and oat bran - Citrus fruits, apples, and pears

- Fruits (strawberries, blueberries) Vegetables (carrots, broccoli, Brussels sprouts) Beans and lentils

4. Insoluble Fiber-Rich Foods:

- Whole grains and whole wheat

- Seeds and nuts, especially while still in their skins Brown rice; vegetables (zucchini, celery, cucumbers); fruit skins (apple, grape, etc.)

• Advice for Including Both Kinds of Fiber:

• In your diet, try to include a range of fruits, vegetables, whole grains, legumes, nuts, and seeds.

• To give your digestive system time to adapt, increase your intake of fiber gradually.

• Because fiber absorbs water and aids in its passage through the digestive system, drink plenty of water.

In addition to promoting general digestive health, a balanced diet that contains a combination of soluble and insoluble fiber can help avoid a number of gastrointestinal problems.

Meal Planning and Recipes

Meal planning for individuals with diverticulitis involves choosing foods that are gentle on the digestive system, low in fiber during flare-ups, and gradually reintroducing high-fiber options during periods of remission. Here are some meal planning tips and simple recipes suitable for individuals with diverticulitis:

Meal Planning Tips:

1. When on a low-fiber diet during flare-ups, select fruits and vegetables that are well-cooked and peeled.

- Choose refined grains such as white bread and rice.

- Add foods high in lean protein, like fish, eggs, and chicken.

- Include dairy products with reduced fat.

- Restrict or stay away from high-fiber meals, seeds, and nuts.

2. During Remission (High-Fiber Diet): Reintroduce whole grains, legumes, fruits, and vegetables that are high in fiber gradually.

• To acquire a spectrum of nutrients, make sure you eat a variety of vibrant fruits and vegetables.

• Add whole grains, such as brown rice, quinoa, and pasta made from whole wheat.

• Include foods high in unsaturated fats, such avocados and olive oil.

• Keep yourself properly hydrated.

Simple Recipes for People with Diverticulitis:

1. Low-Fiber Stir-Fry with Chicken and Vegetables:

Ingredients:

- Skinless, boneless chicken breast
- Sliced and peeled zucchini
- Cooked and sliced carrots

- Low-sodium soy sauce and white rice

- Garlic and ginger for taste

Directions: Stir-fry the chicken until it's done, then add the vegetables and cook until the chicken is soft.

• Add soy sauce, ginger, and garlic for seasoning.

Transfer To White Rice.

2. Low-Fiber Baked Salmon with Mashed Potatoes:

Ingredients:

• Salmon fillets, peeled, boiled, and mashed potatoes, steamed green beans, and olive oil, lemon juice, and herbs for flavor

- **Directions:,** Season salmon with herbs and lemon juice, then bake until done.

- Accompany with steamed green beans and mashed potatoes.

3. High-Fiber Quinoa and Vegetable Salad:

Ingredients: cooked Quinoa

- Diced bell peppers, tomatoes, and cucumbers; canned and washed chickpeas; olive oil and lemon dressing

- **Optional:** Add feta cheese.

- **Directions:** Toss cooked quinoa with chopped veggies and chickpeas.

• Pour some lemon dressing and olive oil on top.

• If preferred, top with crumbled feta cheese.

4. High-Fiber Smoothie Bowl:

Ingredients: Mixed berries (strawberries, blueberries, raspberries) Banana Greek yogurt

• Ground chia or flaxseeds and add honey for sweetness

• **Directions:** Blend banana, Greek yogurt, and berries until smooth.

• Transfer into a bowl and sprinkle chia or ground flaxseeds on top.

• Pour some honey on top for sweetness.

Always consult with a healthcare professional or registered dietitian before making significant changes to your diet, especially if you have diverticulitis or other medical conditions. They can provide personalized advice based on your specific needs and health status.

Cooking Tips for a Healthier Diet

Cooking plays a significant role in promoting a healthier diet, and incorporating certain techniques and choices can enhance the nutritional value of your meals. Here are some cooking tips for a healthier diet:

1. Select Healthier Cooking Techniques: Choose cooking techniques like grilling, baking, steaming, roasting, or sautéing with little oil that call for less additional fats. These techniques aid in maintaining the meals' original flavors and minerals.

2. Use Heart-Healthy Oils: When cooking, use heart-healthy oils like canola, avocado, or olive oil. Because of their high content of monounsaturated fats, these oils may be a preferable option over saturated fats.

3. Use Herbs and Spices to Add Flavor: Experiment with herbs and spices to add flavor instead of depending too much on salt or calorie-dense sauces. Garlic, ginger, fresh herbs, and a range of spices can enhance the flavor and depth of your food without adding unnecessary calories.

4. Use Whole Grains: Use whole grains like barley, brown rice, quinoa, and whole wheat pasta in favor of processed grains. More fiber and nutrients are found in whole grains, which improve digestion and general health.

5. Add a Variety of Veggies: Try to have colorful veggies make up half of your meal. To improve flavors and textures, try experimenting with different cooking techniques like roasting, steaming, or stir-frying.

6. Adopt Lean Proteins: Select lean protein sources such fish, tofu, beans, lentils, and skinless chicken. To lower the total fat level, trim the meat and poultry of any visible fat.

7. Manage Portion Sizes: Pay attention to portion sizes to prevent overindulging. A fuller-looking plate can be achieved by using smaller plates and bowls.

8. Engage in Mindful Eating: Take your time, enjoy every bite, and be aware of your body's signals of hunger and fullness. Better digestion and a reduction in overeating may result from doing this.

9. Reduce Added Sugars: Use as little added sugar as possible in recipes. Instead, use fruits like mashed bananas or berries to organically sweeten food.

10. Make Your Own Sauces and Dressings: Take control of the ingredients and cut back on added sugars, salt, and harmful fats by making your own sauces and dressings.

11. Include Plant-Based Proteins: Increase the amount of plant-based proteins in your meals by include things like nuts, lentils, and beans. These foods offer a range of vital nutrients and are high in fiber.

12. Experiment with Different Cooking Methods: To add diversity to your diet and introduce new textures and flavors, try out new cooking methods like pickling, fermenting, or raw preparation.

13. Remain Hydrated: To stay hydrated, include foods high in water in your meals, like fruits and vegetables. Throughout the day, choose water over sugar-filled drinks.

By adopting these cooking tips, you can create delicious and nutritious meals that support a healthier diet and overall well-being. Remember to enjoy a variety of foods in moderation and consult with a healthcare professional or registered dietitian for personalized advice based on your individual health needs.

CHAPTER FIVE
Hydration and Fluid Intake

Drinking the right amount of fluids and staying hydrated are crucial for general health and wellbeing. Many body processes, such as digestion, nutrition absorption, temperature regulation, and waste removal, depend on maintaining adequate hydration. The following are important guidelines for hydration and fluid intake:

1. Daily Fluid Requirements:

• Age, sex, activity level, climate, and general health are some of the variables that can affect the required daily fluid intake. Generally speaking, though, you should try to consume about 8 cups (64 ounces) of water each day. Particular needs could be greater, particularly during hot weather or when engaging in vigorous exercise.

2. Signs of Dehydration: It's critical to recognize the following symptoms of dehydration:

- Dry lips and skin o Dark yellow urine o Thirst
- Headache
- Fatigue
- Lightheadedness or dizziness

3. Hydration Sources: The main and most effective source of hydration is water. Other drinks that can increase fluid intake include infused water, green tea, and herbal teas. High-water fruits and vegetables, such as oranges, cucumbers, and watermelon, also aid in maintaining hydration.

4. Hydration and Digestive Health: By assisting in the softening of feces and preventing constipation, adequate hydration promotes digestive health. Water is necessary for the digestive system to break down and absorb nutrients.

5. Physical Exercise and Hydration: Physical activity raises the body's fluid requirements. To keep your body hydrated, you must drink water before, during, and after activity.

6. Customizing Fluid Intake: It's important to customize your fluid intake according to your age, weight, activity level, and health condition because each person has different fluid requirements. Women who are nursing or pregnant can need more fluids.

7. Monitoring Urine Color: Keeping an eye on the color of your pee can give you a quick idea of how hydrated you are. While dark yellow or amber urine may indicate dehydration, pale yellow pee often indicates adequate hydration.

8. Factors Affecting Fluid Needs:

• Weather conditions that are hot and muggy can raise the requirement for fluids. Pregnancy, certain drugs, and medical conditions can all affect how much water a person needs.

9. Refraining from Excessive Alcohol and Caffeine: Alcohol and caffeine can have a diuretic effect, which increases urine production and may exacerbate dehydration. It's critical to balance the consumption of these drinks with water.

10. Staying Hydrated All Day: - Aim for steady hydration throughout the day as opposed to guzzling copious amounts of water at once. Drink water on a regular basis to keep your fluid balance stable.

Staying properly hydrated is essential to living a healthy lifestyle. It promotes a number of physiological processes and has a favorable effect on general health. For individualized guidance on fluid consumption, people with particular health problems or conditions should speak with healthcare specialists.

Items to Steer Clear of

Certain foods may need to be restricted or avoided by people with diverticulitis, particularly during flare-ups. Reducing irritation and pressure on the inflamed or infected diverticula is the goal of these recommendations. Remember that everyone has different nutritional requirements, so for individualized advice, speak with a medical practitioner or qualified dietitian. In general, the following foods should be avoided if you have diverticulitis:

1. High-Fiber Foods During Flare-ups: although a high-fiber diet is typically indicated for diverticulosis, it's frequently advised to temporarily restrict fiber consumption during acute flare-ups of diverticulitis. Avoiding fresh fruits and vegetables, nuts, seeds, and whole grains may be part of this.

2. Seeds and Nuts: Seeds and nuts, such as those in whole grains and some fruits, can be irritating and hard to digest. They can also lodge in the diverticula. Whole nuts, pumpkin seeds, and sunflower seeds are a few examples.

3. Popcorn: The hard, tiny kernels in popcorn might cause issues as they can become lodged in the diverticula. Avoiding popcorn is often advised during flare-ups.

4. Specific Raw Fruits and Vegetables: During acute episodes of diverticulitis, raw fruits and vegetables with tough skins or seeds may be difficult to digest. Raw tomatoes, cucumbers, cherries, pears, and apples are a few examples.

5. High-Fat and Spicy Foods: These two dietary categories might aggravate digestive issues. Limiting fried foods, fatty meat cuts, and spicy dishes is advised since they may worsen symptoms.

6. Dairy Products (In Certain Cases): During flare-ups, some people with diverticulitis may become lactose intolerant. It could be wise to minimize dairy products in some situations. Nonetheless, dairy is generally well tolerated by diverticulitis sufferers.

7. Red Meat: Although low protein sources are usually advised, some cuts of red meat may be higher in fat and more difficult to digest than others. Instead, choose lean fish or poultry slices.

8. Refined and Processed Foods: Refined and highly processed foods, such white bread, sugary snacks, and processed meats, should be avoided as they may aggravate inflammation.

9. Alcohol and Caffeine: The digestive system may get irritated by excessive alcohol and caffeine consumption. It's important to practice moderation, and restricting or avoiding alcohol and caffeine during acute bouts may be helpful.

10. Artificial Sweeteners: Some people may experience gastric pain while using certain artificial sweeteners. It could be beneficial to avoid or consume them in moderation.

It's crucial to remember that these are only suggestions; people may respond to particular foods in various ways. It could be advised to follow a low-residue or low-fiber diet when diverticulitis flares up. One option is to gradually reintroduce high-fiber foods when symptoms improve.

A qualified dietician or healthcare expert should always be consulted in order to create a customized eating plan that takes into account each person's preferences, health requirements, and diverticulitis severity.

Modifying Your Lifestyle to Manage Diverticulitis

Diverticulitis management includes dietary modifications as well as lifestyle modifications to support overall digestive health and lower the chance of flare-ups. Those who have diverticulitis may benefit from the following lifestyle modifications:

1. Adopt a High-Fiber Diet: To encourage regular bowel movements, gradually increase your consumption of fiber. Consuming a diet high in fruits, vegetables, whole grains, and legumes can help keep the colon healthy and prevent constipation.

2. Remain Hydrated: To stay properly hydrated, drink a lot of water throughout the day. Staying properly hydrated aids with digestion and helps avoid constipation.

3. Consistent Exercise: Take part in consistent physical activity, such as jogging, swimming, walking, or other exercises. Regular bowel movements and general digestive health are enhanced by exercise.

4. Retain a Healthy Weight: Retaining a healthy weight helps lower the chance of developing diverticulitis and its aftereffects. Regular exercise and a well-balanced diet help in weight management.

5. Give up Smoking: There's evidence linking smoking to a higher risk of diverticulitis. In addition to improving digestive health, quitting smoking has many other positive health effects.

6. Limit Alcohol and Caffeine: It is best to consume alcohol and caffeinated drinks in moderation as too much of either might aggravate the digestive tract.

7. Handle Stress: Prolonged stress might have an impact on digestive health. Include stress-reduction strategies in your routine, such as yoga, deep breathing exercises, meditation, or other relaxation techniques.

8. Regular Bowel Routines: Create and preserve regular routines for your bowels. To maintain a healthy digestive rhythm, try to keep mealtimes and restroom breaks at regular times.

9. Use of Nonsteroidal Anti-Inflammatory Drugs (NSAIDs) Should Be Limited: Extended use of NSAIDs, including ibuprofen, may raise the risk of diverticulitis. See your healthcare practitioner about other options if you require pain relief.

10. Comply with Medical Advice: Take prescription drugs as instructed by your physician. Infections related to diverticulitis may require the use of antibiotics.

11. Regular Health Checkups: Make an appointment for routine examinations with your physician to keep an eye on your general health and to quickly address any issues or symptoms.

12. Recognize Triggers: Keep an eye out for meals or lifestyle choices that can aggravate symptoms. To help you locate probable triggers, keep a food journal. Share your results with your healthcare professional.

13. Take Probiotics Into Account: Probiotics, which include good microorganisms, may assist intestinal health. Have a conversation with your healthcare practitioner about using probiotics.

It's important to remember that everyone reacts differently to changes in lifestyle. See a medical expert for tailored guidance based on your unique health status, symptoms, and requirements. Maintaining good contact with your medical team is essential to managing diverticulitis effectively.

Medication and Supplements

Certain vitamins and drugs may be used to treat diverticulitis, but it's crucial to remember that any use of vitamins or drugs should be discussed with and prescribed by a healthcare provider. The following are a few popular vitamins and drugs for diverticulitis:

1. Antibiotics: In cases where diverticulitis is linked to an infection, a prescription for antibiotics may be necessary to address the bacterial inflammation. Antibiotics like ciprofloxacin, metronidazole, and amoxicillin-clavulanate are frequently utilized.

2. Pain Management Products:

• Because of the possibility of exacerbating symptoms or consequences, nonsteroidal anti-inflammatory medicines (NSAIDs), such ibuprofen or naproxen, are often avoided during acute episodes of diverticulitis. It might be advised to take acetaminophen to relieve pain.

3. Fiber Supplements: To help maintain regular bowel movements and prevent constipation, healthcare practitioners may suggest fiber supplements during periods of remission. Supplements with psyllium husk are a popular option.

4. Probiotics: Supplements containing advantageous bacteria can assist maintain a balanced and healthy population of gut flora. Some people find that taking probiotics on a daily basis helps them feel better. On the other hand, research is currently ongoing to determine their effectiveness in treating diverticulitis.

5. Bulk-Forming Agents: These substances, such psyllium or methylcellulose, can assist increase the volume of the stool and encourage frequent bowel motions. During times of remission, they are frequently utilized as a preventative strategy.

6. Pain Management Drugs: During acute bouts, prescription painkillers may be suggested to treat severe pain. These are usually used under a healthcare provider's supervision for a brief period of time.

7. Drugs for Bowel Spasms:

• Antispasmodic drugs, including dicyclomine, may be recommended to treat the symptoms of stomach pain and bowel spasms.

8. Immunomodulators and Biologics: Immunomodulators or biologic drugs may be investigated to modify the immune response and reduce inflammation in certain situations, especially if the diverticulitis is severe or recurrent. This is less frequent and typically used in instances that are more complex.

Diverticulitis patients must collaborate closely with their medical professionals to identify the best course of action for their specific needs, medical history, and degree of symptoms. Self-medication or taking supplements without consulting a doctor can result in side effects or inadequate results.

The total strategy for treating diverticulitis should also include lifestyle adjustments including eating better, getting regular exercise, and reducing stress. Always heed the advice of your healthcare practitioner, and report any new or worsening symptoms right once.

Conclusion

Finally, it should be noted that diverticulitis is a disorder marked by inflammation or infection of tiny pouches (diverticula) that may form in the colon's walls. Diverticulitis can cause symptoms including abdominal pain, tenderness, and changes in bowel habits, but diverticulosis, or the presence of diverticula, is common and frequently asymptomatic.

• Diverticulitis is treated with a mix of dietary adjustments, lifestyle alterations, and, occasionally, medication. Diverticulosis is usually prevented and managed with high-fiber diets; however, low-fiber or low-residue diets may be suggested during acute flare-ups. Maintaining a healthy weight, exercising frequently, and drinking plenty of water are all crucial for maintaining digestive health.

• During acute episodes, some foods, such seeds, nuts, and high-fiber goods, may need to be restricted, and it's important to stay away from known triggers. Modest alcohol and caffeine use, stress management, and stopping smoking are examples of lifestyle modifications that support a comprehensive approach to diverticulitis treatment.

• Certain symptoms or consequences may require the prescription of drugs such probiotics, antibiotics, analgesics, and fiber supplements. Diverticulitis sufferers should collaborate closely with medical providers to create a treatment plan that is specific to their requirements and condition.

• Crucial components of the continuing therapy of diverticulitis include routine examinations, symptom monitoring, and following prescription guidelines. It can be essential to undergo more medical testing and, in certain situations, surgery if problems develop or the symptoms don't go away.

Diverticulitis can cause different symptoms in different people, just like any other medical disease, so getting expert advice is crucial. For an accurate diagnosis and course of treatment, it is imperative that you seek medical attention as soon as you suspect you may have diverticulitis or notice any symptoms.

THE END